Dr. J's
ECG in
a Day

Best Aid Reviews
Mohsen Javaheri, MD

Dr. J's
ECG
in a Day

Mohsen Javaheri, MD
Copyright © 2024 by BEST AID REVIEWS

Notice

Contents

Preface

Welcome to "Dr. J's ECG in a Day." This concise guide is designed to quickly demystify electrocardiography for students, new healthcare professionals, and anyone interested in understanding the heart's electrical signals.

Electrocardiography is essential in diagnosing and monitoring heart conditions, offering a non-invasive peek into the heart's electrical activity. Despite its clinical importance, the art of ECG interpretation can seem overwhelming due to its complex patterns and nuances.

This book simplifies ECG interpretation by starting with the basics of heart anatomy and electrical physiology, then progresses to reading and understanding ECG strips, and recognizing key indicators of cardiac health and disease.

Structured to facilitate rapid learning, "Dr. J's ECG in a Day" is filled with practical examples and essential knowledge to boost your confidence in interpreting ECGs effectively. Let's embark on this fast-paced educational journey to unlock the secrets of the heart's electrical language.

Chapter 1

The Basics of ECG

Introduction

Electrocardiography records the electrical activity of the heart. The heart has an electrical system with wiring that maintains the normal rhythm.

Electrical activity of the heart

The heart's rhythmic contractions are initiated by electrical impulses generated by the sinoatrial (SA) node, located in the right atrium. This "natural pacemaker" sets the pace for the heart rate.

The electrical impulse from the SA node spreads through the atria, leading to their contraction, and then travels to the atrioventricular (AV) node.

After a brief delay at the AV node, which allows the ventricles to fill with blood, the impulse travels down the His–Purkinje system (the heart's electrical wiring), causing the ventricles to contract and pump blood to the lungs and the rest of the body.

The bundle of His splits into the right and left bundle branches along the interventricular septum (the wall separating the left and right ventricles)

The left bundle branch itself divides into the anterior and posterior fascicles, which help ensure that the large, muscular left ventricle contracts in a coordinated manner.

The branches distribute the impulse to the Purkinje fibers, which spread throughout the ventricular walls. This network ensures rapid and coordinated contraction of the ventricles, which pump blood out to the lungs and the rest of the body.

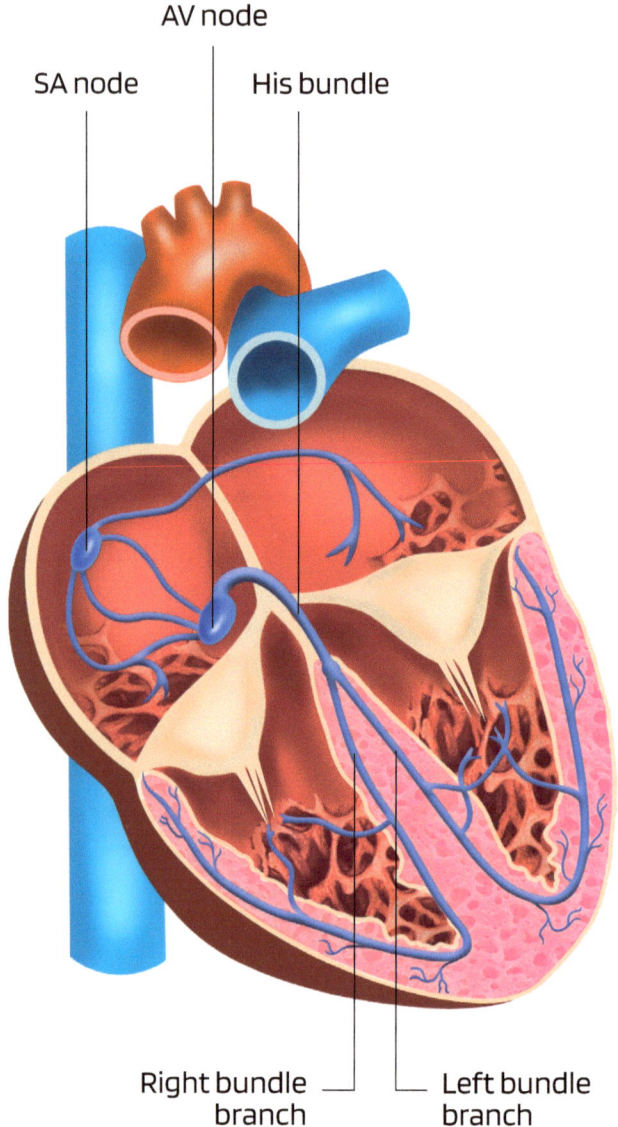

Conduction pathways

The signal travels from the SA node to the AV node. After a delay in the AV node, the signal is transmitted to the His bundle, then to right and left bundle branches. Finally the signal travels to the purkinje fibers.

The principles behind ECG recording

An ECG machine, using skin electrodes, records and amplifies the heart's electrical activity by measuring the voltage differences generated by this electrical flow across the heart muscle.

The resulting tracing reflects the sequence of depolarization and repolarization of the atria and ventricles.

Depolarization corresponds to muscle contraction, while repolarization corresponds to muscle relaxation. The main components of the ECG tracing are the P wave, QRS complex, and T wave, each representing different phases of the heart's electrical cycle.

Overview of ECG machine and setup

An ECG machine typically consists of a set of leads (electrical cables) that connect to electrodes. These electrodes are strategically placed on the patient's limbs and chest to capture the heart's electrical activity from various angles. The standard ECG uses 12 leads, generated from 10 physical electrodes, to produce 12 different electrical views of the heart.

The placement of these electrodes is crucial for accurate interpretation of the ECG. Incorrect placement can lead to misinterpretation of the heart's electrical activity, potentially resulting in a misdiagnosis. Therefore, understanding the correct setup is the first practical step in learning to perform and interpret ECGs.

A normal ECG with 12 leads includes three unipolar leads, three augmented leads, and six precordial leads.

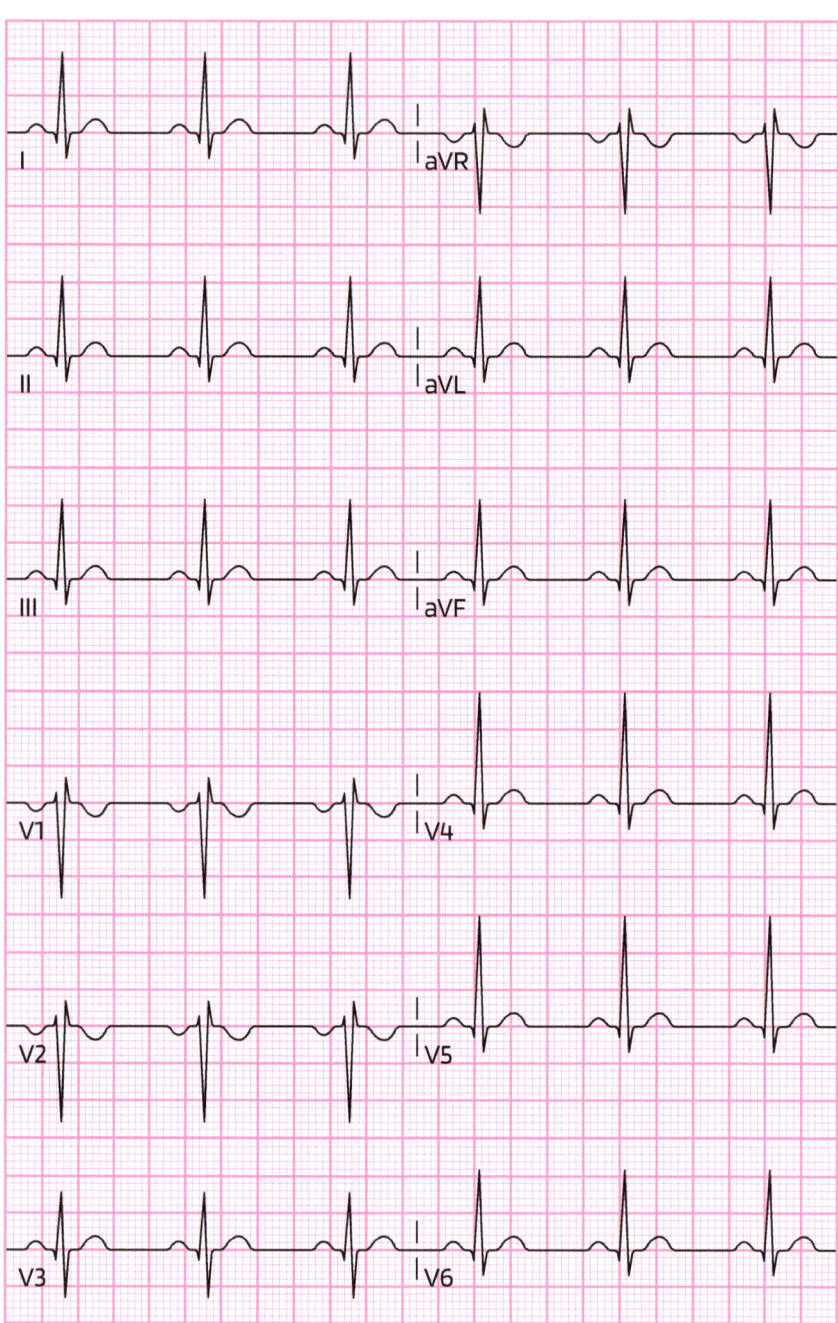

Normal 12-lead ECG

Bipolar leads

Bipolar leads are lead I, lead II, and lead III.

>   **Lead I**: Measures the electrical potential between the right arm (negative electrode) and the left arm (positive electrode). This lead shows the heart's electrical activity from the right side toward the left.

>   **Lead II**: Measures the electrical potential between the right arm (negative electrode) and the left leg (positive electrode). This lead provides a view of the heart's electrical activity from the right shoulder diagonally down to the left leg, which is particularly useful for assessing the heart's rhythm.

>   **Lead III**: Measures the electrical potential between the left arm (negative electrode) and the left leg (positive electrode). This lead offers a view from the left side of the body to the left leg.

When you join these three leads together, they form the Einthoven triangle.
So we have three bipolar leads, three unipolar leads, and six precordial leads. The 3 bipolar leads make the Einthoven triangle.

The 3 **unipolar limb leads** are aVL, aVF, and aVR.
> AVL: oriented at at -30 degrees
> aVF: oriented at 90 degrees
> aVR: oriented is at -150 degrees.

The **precordial leads** consist of six leads, named V1 through V6, each placed in specific locations on the chest:
> **V1**: 4th intercostal space, just to the right of the sternum.
> **V2**: 4th intercostal space, just to the left of the sternum.
> **V3**: Between leads V2 and V4
> **V4**: 5th intercostal space at the midclavicular line.
> **V5**: Horizontally in line with V4 at the left anterior axillary line.
> **V6**: Horizontally in line with V4 and V5 at the left midaxillary line.

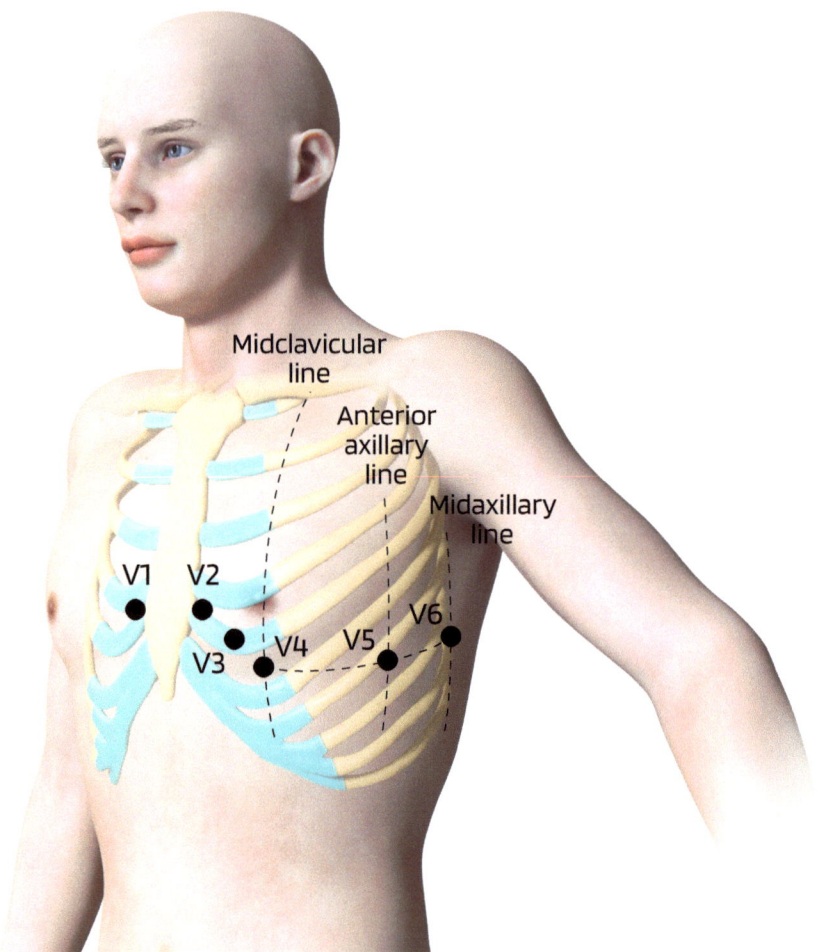

Midclavicular line

Anterior axillary line

Midaxillary line

V1 V2

V3 V4 V5 V6

Precordial leads

The positions of the precordial leads are shown.

Chapter 2
Reading ECG strips

Introduction to the ECG paper and measurements

An ECG strip is printed on graph paper marked by small and large squares. Understanding the significance of these squares is crucial for accurate measurement and interpretation:

> **Small squares**: Each small square on the ECG paper represents 0.04 seconds horizontally, and 0.1 mV in voltage vertically.

> **Large squares**: Each large square is made up of 5x5 small squares, representing 0.2 seconds horizontally and 0.5 mV vertically.

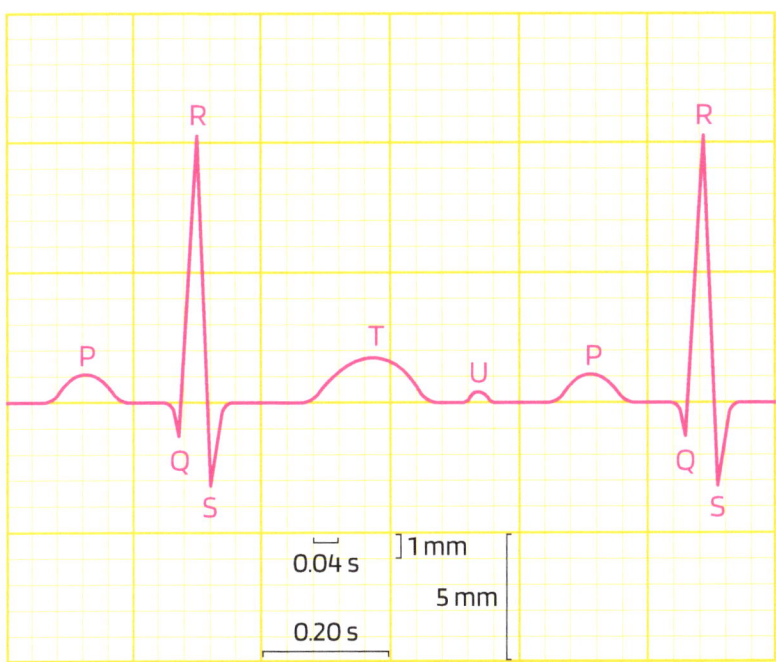

ECG strip with small and large boxes

The positions of the unipolar and augmented leads can be visualized as being arranged in a circle, with each lead providing a unique angle of view of the heart's electrical activity. The angles of these leads are shown here:

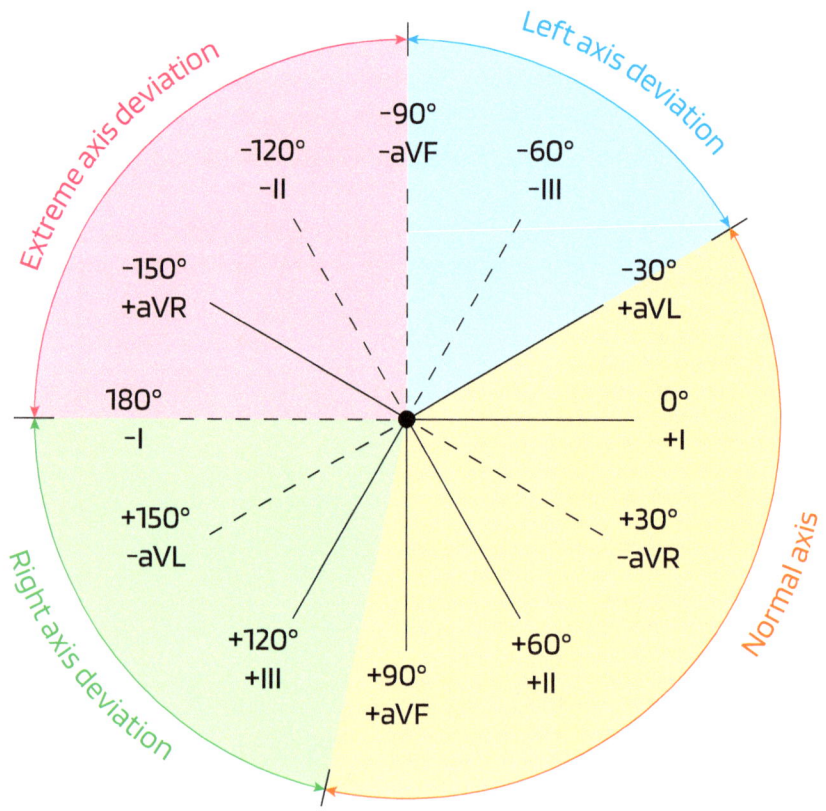

Unipolar and bipolar leads

The standard speed at which the paper moves through an ECG machine is 25 mm/sec. This consistent speed makes time and rate calculations straightforward once you are familiar with the grid system.

Basic rhythm interpretation

To interpret an ECG rhythm, begin by identifying the following components on the strip:

> **P wave**: Represents atrial depolarization. A normal P wave is smooth, rounded, and upright in most leads, and it precedes each QRS complex.

> **QRS complex**: Represents ventricular depolarization. It normally lasts 0.08 to 0.12 seconds. A QRS duration greater than 0.12 seconds suggests a delay in ventricular conduction.

> **T wave**: Represents ventricular repolarization. It is normally smooth and rounded, with a direction generally the same as the QRS complex.

> **PR interval**: Measures the time from the beginning of the P wave to the start of the QRS complex, indicating the time the electrical impulse takes to travel from the sinus node through the AV node. The normal PR interval ranges from 0.12 to 0.20 seconds.

> **QT interval**: Measures the duration of ventricular depolarization and repolarization, from the start of the QRS complex to the end of the T wave. The normal QT interval varies based on the heart rate and should be corrected for rate (QTc).

The significance of intervals and segments

> **PR interval**: As mentioned, it represents the time it takes for the electrical impulse to travel from the atria to the ventricles. A prolonged PR interval may indicate first-degree heart block, while a shortened PR interval may be seen in conditions like Wolff-Parkinson-White syndrome.

> **ST segment**: The segment between the end of the S wave and the start of the T wave is the ST segment, representing the period between ventricular depolarization and repolarization. **ST elevation** or **ST depression** can indicate myocardial infarction or ischemia.

> **Identifying Heart Rate**: To calculate the heart rate on an ECG strip, count the number of QRS complexes in a 6-second strip and multiply by 10. Alternatively, for regular rhythms, you can calculate the rate by measuring the distance between R waves in large squares and then dividing 300 by the number of large squares between R waves.

Characteristics of a normal ECG reading

A normal ECG displays certain key features that indicate the heart's electrical activity is functioning correctly. These features include:

> **P wave**: The initial deflection, representing atrial depolarization, appears before each QRS complex. It should be upright in most leads, except for aVR, where it is normally inverted.

> **QRS complex**: Follows the P wave and represents ventricular depolarization. It should be narrow, typically less than 0.12 seconds (or 3 small squares in duration, indicating efficient conduction through the ventricles.

> **T wave**: Reflects ventricular repolarization and follows the QRS complex. It should be upright in most leads, mirroring the direction of the QRS complex in that lead.

> **PR interval**: Ranging from 0.12 to 0.20 seconds (3 to 5 small squares), this interval indicates the time from the beginning of atrial depolarization to the beginning of ventricular depolarization.

> **QT interval**: The duration from the start of the QRS complex to the end of the T wave is known as the QT interval. It varies with heart rate but is typically less than half the preceding R–R interval at normal heart rates.

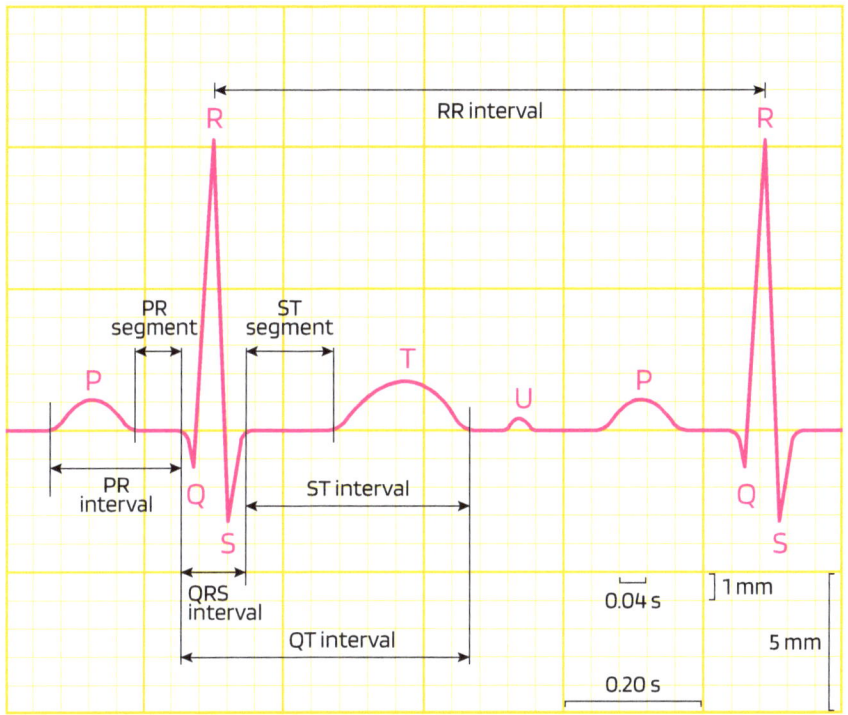

Charactersitics of a normal ECG beat

Heart rate calculation

The heart rate can be determined by measuring the interval between two consecutive QRS complexes. A simple method for calculating the heart rate on a standard ECG, where the paper speed is 25 mm/second, is the "300 rule." Count the number of large squares between two R waves and divide 300 by this number. The result is the approximate heart rate per minute.

Axis determination

The electrical axis of the heart refers to the general direction of the heart's electrical depolarization. It is calculated using the limb leads. A normal axis falls between –30° and +110°. Determining the heart's electrical axis can provide insights into various cardiac conditions.

The heart axis can be determined by examining two leads: lead I and aVF.

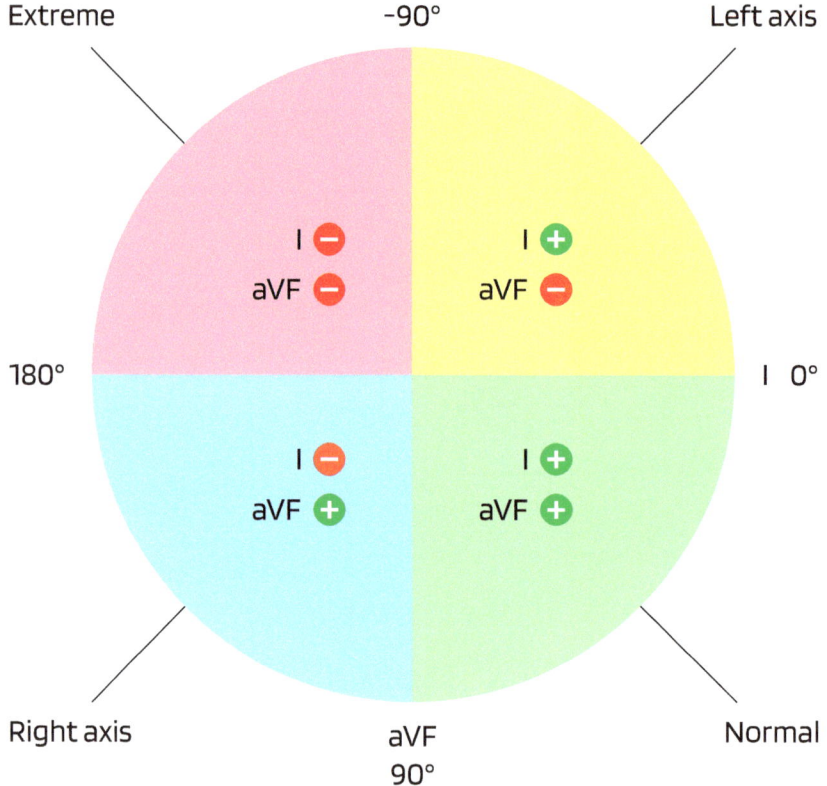

Determining the heart axis

This method can determine the majority of the cases of axis deviation.

> First, the sum of the QRS complex in lead I and aVF is measured. The sum means adding up all positive and negative deflections of the Q, R, and S waves.

> If the sum of the QRS complexes in both of these leads is positive, then the heart axis falls between zero degrees and 90 degrees. This indicates a normal heart axis.

> If the sum of the QRS complexes is negative in lead I and is positive in aVF then it is between 90 and 180 degrees, which is considered **right axis deviation** in the majority of cases.

> If the sum is positive in lead I and negative in aVF then it falls between 0 degrees and –90 degrees, which is considered **left axis deviation** in the majority of cases.

> In the case that the sum of QRS complexes is negative in both lead I and lead aVF, then it is considered **extreme axis deviation**, which could be caused by an initial right or left axis deviation.

> **Left axis deviation**: This may indicate left ventricular hypertrophy or a conduction block.

> **Right axis deviation**: This may suggest right ventricular hypertrophy, chronic lung disease, or a conduction block.

Summary of how to read ECG strips

In a systematic approach, first ensure that there are no technical errors. If everything looks unusually large or small, double-check to see if the calibration is correct and if the limb electrodes are connected properly.

Rate and rhythm

If the R-R intervals are equal, the heart rate can be determined by dividing 300 by the number of large boxes between the R-R intervals. If the R-R intervals are not equal, count the number of QRS complexes in the strip and multiply by 6 (assuming the strip duration is 10 seconds).

This method is particularly useful in cases of atrial fibrillation and multifocal atrial tachycardia, where the R-R intervals change constantly. If the number of 5 mm boxes (large boxes) between R-R waves is between 3-5, the heart rate is normal. More than 5 boxes indicate bradycardia, while fewer than 3 boxes indicate tachycardia. A normal heart rate ranges between 60 and 100 beats per minute. For reference, dividing 300 by 5 boxes results in 60 beats per minute, and dividing 300 by 3 boxes results in 100 beats per minute.

Rule out technical errors	Double check the position of leads and calibration
Rate	300 divided by the number of 5 mm boxes
Rhythm	Make sure it is sinus by checking P waves before every QRS
P wave	Atrial hypertrophy (large P wave) & atrial fibrillation (lack of P waves)
PR interval & AV blocks	Normal value is 0.12 – 0.20
QRS interval, axis & voltage	Wide QRS is seen in bundle branch block & hypertrophy
QT interval	Corrected QT interval is more reliable (QT/√RR) and should be ≤440 milliseconds
Q wave, ST segments & T waves	Rule out ischemic heart diseases
U wave	Hypokalemia

Summary of steps how to read ECG

Waves

The **P wave** represents atrial polarization.

The **QRS wave** represents ventricular depolarization.

The **T wave** represents ventricular repolarization. Atrial repolarization is not seen on ECG as it is embedded within the QRS complex.

Occasionally, a **U wave** may appear after the T wave in some normal subjects. However, the presence of a prominent U wave is usually a sign of hypokalemia.

P pulmonale refers to a P wave in lead II that is over 2.5 millimeters in height, indicating right atrial hypertrophy. This is significant because the height of the P wave reaches or exceeds half of a large box on the ECG grid. Each small box represents 0.04 seconds, and each large box (comprising five small boxes) represents 0.20 seconds.

P mitrale is characterized by a notched P wave and is a sign of left atrial hypertrophy.

A **Q wave** must be more than 0.04 seconds in duration to potentially indicate a transmural infarction. It is typically a late sign of myocardial infarction.

The **T wave** represents ventricular repolarization. A negative T wave can be a sign of ischemia.

Segments and intervals

An interval includes a wave. For example, the PR interval includes the P wave and the PR segment. The PR segment is specifically the flat line between the end of the P wave and the start of the QRS complex.

Similarly, the ST segment is the flat line between the end of the QRS complex and the start of the T wave. It begins at the end of the S wave and ends at the beginning of the T wave.

The **PR interval** represents the delay at the AV node, which allows time for the atria to contract and fill the ventricles with blood before ventricular contraction.

The **QT interval** encompasses the entire process of ventricular depolarization and repolarization. It is a crucial measurement for assessing the overall electrical activity of the ventricles.

The **ST segment** starts from the end of the S wave and extends to the beginning of the T wave. This segment is extremely important in diagnosing cardiac conditions:

ST elevation is a sign of myocardial infarction (heart attack).

ST depression indicates myocardial ischemia or angina pectoris.

Left ventricular hypertrophy (LVH) is suspected when there are tall R waves and deep S waves. A common criterion for LVH is the sum of the S wave in V1 and the R wave in V5 or V6 being more than 35 millimeters (more than 35 small boxes).

Right ventricular hypertrophy (RVH) is suspected if there is right axis deviation. One criterion for RVH is an R wave in V1 that is more than 7 millimeters. There are other criteria for determining RVH and LVH, but these are among the most commonly used.

The steps in reading an ECG can vary among physicians. The most important rule is to follow a systematic approach to ensure no important information is missed. It is worth noting that in the case of acute chest pain, the first priority is to rule out myocardial ischemia or infarction.

Chapter 3
Arrhythmias

Arrhythmias, or abnormal heart rhythms, are among the most critical conditions detected by ECG. They can range from benign to life-threatening. Understanding the ECG patterns associated with different arrhythmias is essential for accurate diagnosis and management. This chapter explores common arrhythmias, their ECG characteristics, and their clinical significance.

Overview of common arrhythmias

Arrhythmias can be broadly classified into bradyarrhythmias (heart rate <60/min), tachyarrhythmias (heart rate >100/min), and irregular rhythms. They can originate in the atria or ventricles and may affect the heart's efficiency in pumping blood.

Premature atrial contraction (PAC)

A signal from the SA node or an atrial fiber enters earlier than usual, causing the next beat to appear with a small delay as the SA node tries to maintain the same heart rate. Premature atrial contractions (PACs) may present as palpitations or anxiety; however, they are typically benign.

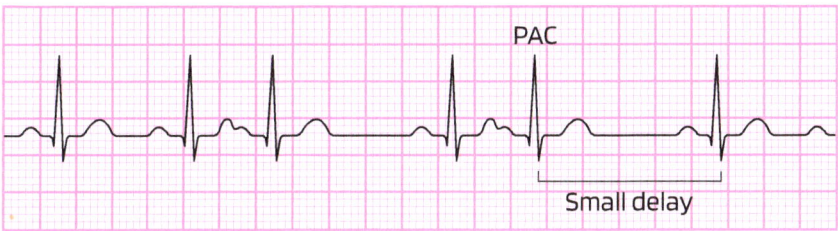

Premature atrial contraction

Premature ventricular contraction (PVC)

A signal from the ventricular fibers takes over the command of the heart, resulting in an early beat. The next signal comes with a small delay as the SA node attempts to maintain the same heart rate. The difference between a premature atrial contraction (PAC) and a premature ventricular contraction (PVC) lies in their shapes. A PVC has a wide QRS complex because the direction of depolarization is from the ventricles upwards. Three consecutive PVCs are considered ventricular tachycardia.

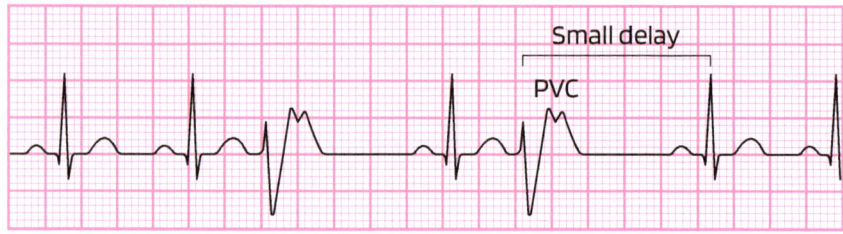

Premature ventricular contraction

Supraventricular tachycardias
Sinus tachycardia

When the heart rate is above 100 beats per minute and the P wave is seen before every QRS complex, with the QRS complex appearing narrow and normal, it is called sinus tachycardia. Sinus tachycardia can be seen in conditions such as fever, pain, infection, exercise, hyperthyroidism, and hypovolemia. It is a very common finding in hospitalized patients.

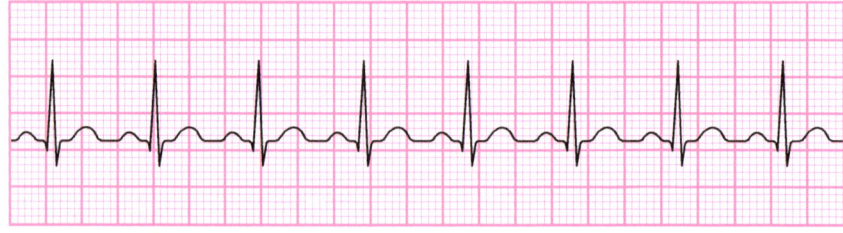

Sinus tachycardia

Atrial fibrillation (AFib)

ECG characteristics: Absent P waves; irregularly irregular R-R intervals; and a variable ventricular response. The baseline may show fine or coarse fibrillatory waves.

Clinical significance: AFib increases the risk of stroke and heart failure. Management may include rate control, rhythm control, and anticoagulation to prevent thromboembolic events.

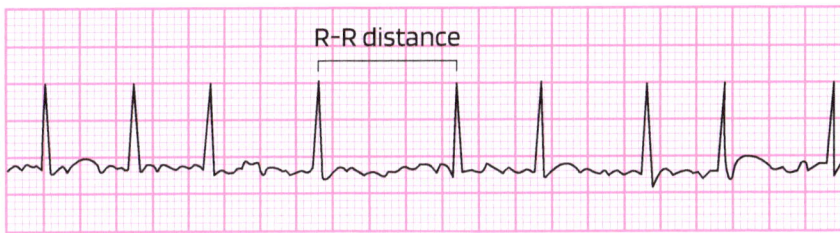

R-R distance

Atrial fibrillation

Atrial flutter

ECG characteristics: Sawtooth-like flutter waves, especially noticeable in leads II, III, and aVF. Typically, a regular ventricular response if there is a fixed block (e.g., 2:1, 3:1).If the atrial rate is 300 bpm and there is a 2:1 conduction, the ventricular rate is 150 bpm. If there is a 3:1 conduction, the heart rate is 75 bpm.

Clinical significance: Atrial flutter can lead to significant hemodynamic compromise and shares a stroke risk similar to atrial fibrillation (AFib), requiring similar management strategies.

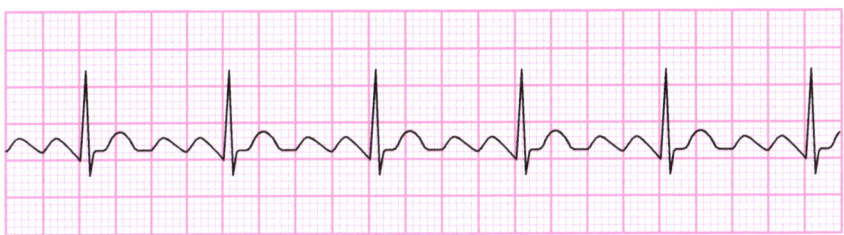

Atrial flutter

Multifocal atrial tachycardia

ECG characteristics: The heart rate is typically over 100 beats per minute.In multifocal atrial tachycardia (MAT), each beat has a differently shaped P wave. The R–R intervals vary, but the presence of P waves differentiates MAT from atrial fibrillation.

Clinical significance: Multifocal atrial tachycardia is strongly associated with COPD.

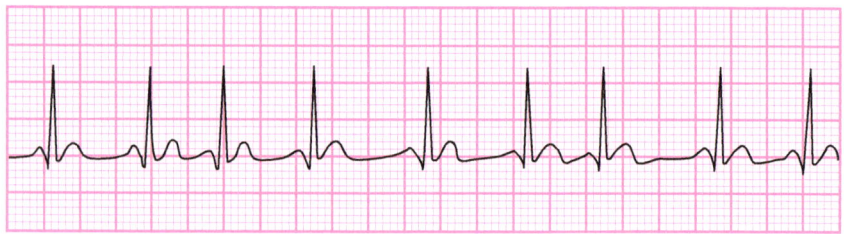

Multifocal atrial tachycardia

Junctional tachycardia

This is a narrow QRS complex tachycardia, that originates from the AV junction (AV node and the area around it).

P waves: P waves may be absent, inverted, or occur just before, during, or after the QRS complex, depending on the exact site of origin within the AV junction and the timing of atrial activation relative to ventricular activation.

QRS complexes:The QRS complexes are usually narrow and normal in duration unless there is a coexisting bundle branch block, as the ventricles are typically activated through the normal conduction system.

Rate: The heart rate in junctional tachycardia is elevated but usually not as rapid as in some forms of supraventricular tachycardia (SVT), such as atrial fibrillation or atrial flutter.

Causes

> **Heart surgery:** It's particularly common in children after surgery for congenital heart disease.

> **Drug toxicity:** Medications like digoxin can increase the risk.
> **Myocardial infarction:** Damage to the heart tissue can lead to arrhythmias, including junctional tachycardia.
> **Electrolyte imbalances:** Abnormal levels of potassium, magnesium, or calcium can contribute to the development of this condition.

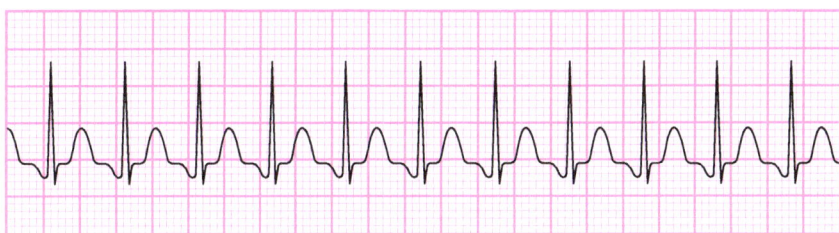

Junctional tachycardia

Paroxysmal supraventricular tachycardia (SVT)

ECG characteristics: A narrow complex tachycardia (QRS duration <0.12 seconds) with a heart rate typically greater than 150 bpm.
P waves may be buried within the QRS complex or appear after it.
Clinical significance: Supraventricular tachycardia (SVT) can cause distressing palpitations for the patient but is generally not life-threatening.Treatment options include vagal maneuvers, medications, and, in some cases, electrophysiological studies and ablation.

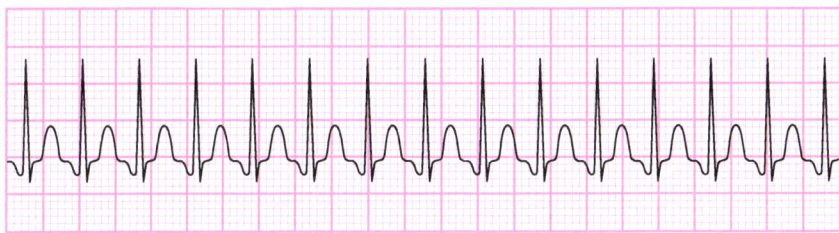

Paroxysmal supraventricular tachycardia

Ventricular tachyarrhythmias
Ventricular tachycardia (VT)

ECG characteristics: A series of three or more QRS complexes occurring at a rate of more than 100 beats per minute. The QRS complex is wide (>0.12 seconds) and often has a bizarre appearance.

Clinical significance: Ventricular tachycardia (VT) can be stable or unstable and has the potential to deteriorate into ventricular fibrillation, a life-threatening condition requiring immediate intervention, such as defibrillation.

Pulseless ventricular tachycardia is treated as cardiopulmonary arrest and requires immediate cardiopulmonary resuscitation (CPR).

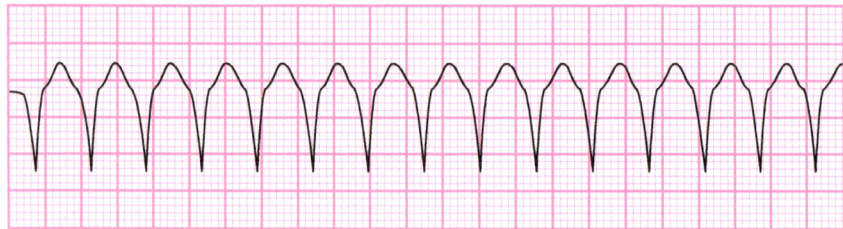

Ventricular tachycardia

Torsades de Pointes

Torsades de Pointes is a unique form of polymorphic ventricular tachycardia characterized by a gradual change in the amplitude and twisting of the QRS complexes around the isoelectric line on the ECG. This distinctive pattern resembles the twisting points of a French braid. The name "Torsades de Pointes" is French for "twisting of the points."

Characteristics of Torsades de Pointes:
> **Rate:** Rapid heart rate, usually between 200 and 250 beats per minute.
> **Rhythm:** The QRS complex amplitude varies, giving the appearance of a twisting pattern. The polarity of the QRS complexes appears to twist back and forth around the baseline.
> **Duration:** Episodes can be brief and self-terminating, or they can persist and progress to ventricular fibrillation, a life-threatening condition.

Causes
TdP is often associated with a prolonged QT interval, which may be caused by:

> **Congenital long QT syndromes:** Genetic conditions leading to prolonged repolarization.

> **Acquired causes:** Certain medications, electrolyte imbalances (especially low levels of potassium or magnesium), and bradycardia can prolong the QT interval and potentially lead to TdP. Examples of medications that prolong the QT interval include:
Antiarrhythmics: Amiodarone, Sotalol
Antibiotics: Azithromycin, Levofloxacin
Antipsychotics: Haloperidol, Quetiapine
Antidepressants: Citalopram, Escitalopram
Others: Methadone, Ondansetron

> **Other factors:** Heart diseases and toxins can also contribute.

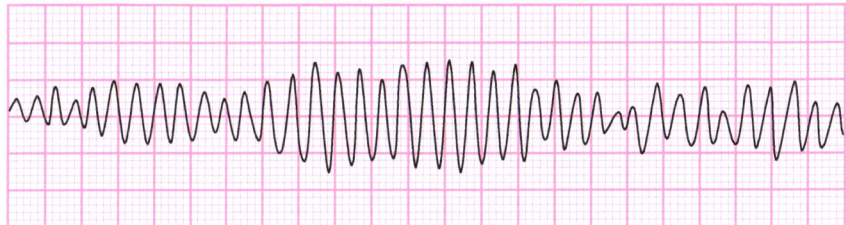

Torsades de Pointes

Ventricular fibrillation

Ventricular fibrillation is a severe cardiac rhythm disturbance characterized by rapid, erratic electrical impulses that cause the ventricles (the heart's lower chambers) to quiver ineffectively instead of pumping blood. This results in the cessation of blood flow to the body, leading to collapse and sudden cardiac death if not treated immediately. By definition, ventricular fibrillation requires immediate cardiopulmonary resuscitation (CPR) and defibrillation.

ECG characteristics

> No discernible P waves, QRS complexes, or T waves.
> Extremely irregular and chaotic electrical activity, with varying amplitude and frequency, appearing as a wavy baseline on the ECG.
> Absence of an identifiable pattern or rhythm.

Causes

VF can be triggered by various factors, including:

> Acute myocardial infarction (heart attack).
> Ischemia (lack of blood supply to the heart muscle).
> Cardiomyopathy (disease of the heart muscle).
> Electrolyte imbalances, particularly potassium and magnesium abnormalities.
> Drug toxicity or overdose (e.g., antiarrhythmic drugs, cocaine).
> Electrical shock or severe trauma.
> Hypothermia.

Symptoms

> Sudden collapse.
> Loss of consciousness.
> Absence of pulse and breathing.
> Death, if not promptly treated.

Treatment

Immediate treatment is crucial for survival and includes:

> **Cardiopulmonary resuscitation (CPR):** Provides temporary artificial blood flow to the brain and vital organs until defibrillation can be performed.

> **Defibrillation:** The application of an electric shock to the chest to restore a normal heart rhythm. This is the most effective treatment for VF and is typically performed with an automated external defibrillator (AED) or in a hospital setting.

> **Advanced cardiac life support (ACLS):** Following initial resuscitation efforts, medications (e.g., epinephrine, antiarrhythmic drugs) and further interventions may be necessary as part of ACLS protocols.

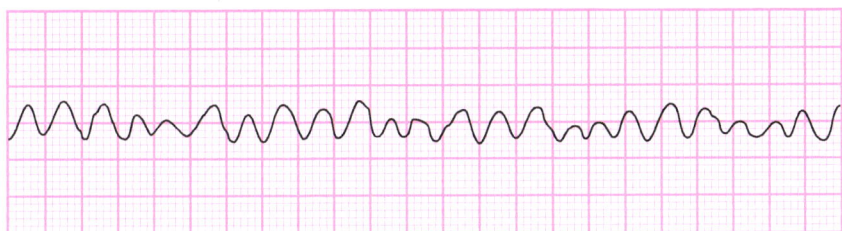

Ventricular fibrillation

Bradyarrhythmia and AV blocks
Sinus bradycardia

ECG characteristics: A heart rate of less than 60 bpm with a P wave before every QRS represents sinus bradycardia, which may be associated with a normal finding in athletes or indicate pathological sinus node dysfunction.

Clinical significance: Pathological bradycardia can lead to inadequate cardiac output and symptoms of fatigue, dizziness, or syncope. Treatment depends on symptoms and may include a pacemaker.

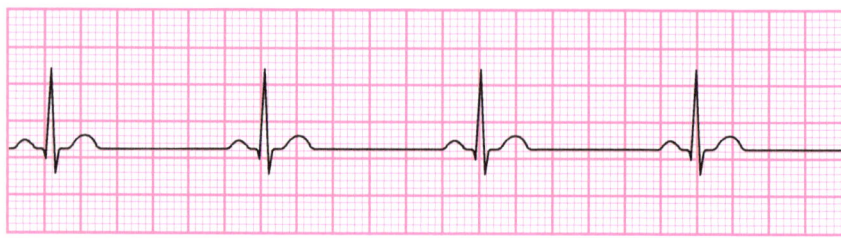

Sinus bradycardia

AV blocks

Atrioventricular (AV) blocks are a group of disorders characterized by a delay or interruption in the electrical communication between the atria and ventricles. This disturbance occurs at the AV node or in the bundle branches that lead to the ventricles. There are three primary types of AV block, distinguished by their severity and ECG characteristics:

First-degree AV block

ECG findings: Prolonged PR interval (greater than 0.20 seconds) but each P wave is followed by a QRS complex.

Clinical significance: Often asymptomatic and may be found incidentally on an ECG. It can be seen in healthy individuals, particularly athletes, or associated with conditions like myocarditis, certain medications, or ischemic heart disease.

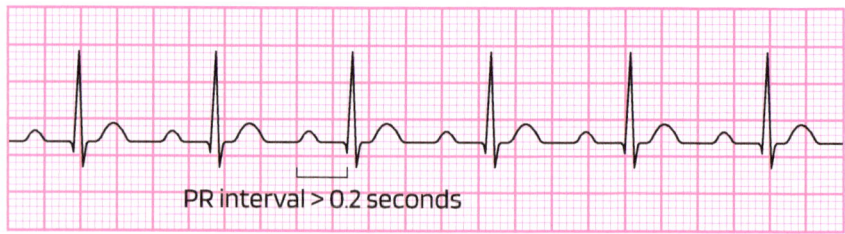

PR interval > 0.2 seconds

First degree heart block

Second-degree AV block

This is further divided into two types:

> **Type I (Mobitz I/Wenckebach):** Progressive prolongation of the PR interval until a beat QRS complex) is dropped. T, which means a P wave is not followed by a QRS complex. The cycle then repeats. Clinical Significance: Often benign and may not require treatment if asymptomatic. It is usually due to reversible causes like increased vagal tone or medications.

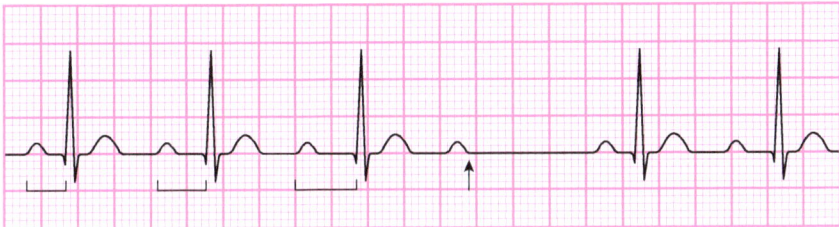

Second-degree heart block type I (Wenckebach)

> **Type II (Mobitz II):** Fixed PR interval with occasional dropped QRS complexes. This is more serious than Type I. It is caused by structural damage to the conductions system of the heart and may require a pacemaker as it can progress to a complete heart block.

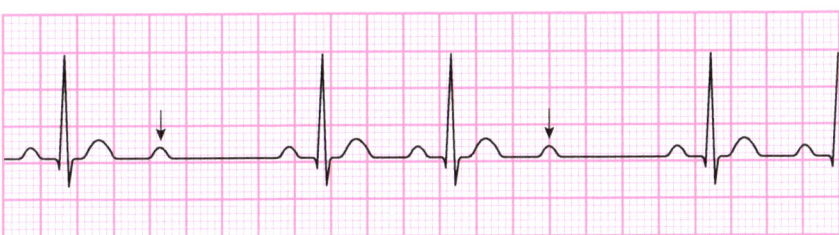

Second-degree heart block type II

Third-degree (complete) AV block

In third-degree heart block, the atria and the vetricles are divorced and work separately without any connection to each other.

ECG findings

Atria and ventricles beat independently of each other. P waves with a regular atrial rhythm and QRS complexes with a slower and different regular rhythm. There is no relationship between the P waves and QRS complexes (atrioventricular dissociation).

Clinical significance

This is a medical emergency if it causes symptoms like syncope, heart failure, or shock. It often requires the urgent placement of a pacemaker.

Treatment

First-degree AV block: May not require any treatment if asymptomatic.

Second-degree AV block (Wenckebach): Often does not require treatment if asymptomatic.

Second-degree AV block (Mobitz II): Typically necessitates cemaker implantation.

Third-degree AV block: Requires pacemaker implantation to maintain an adequate heart rate and prevent symptoms.

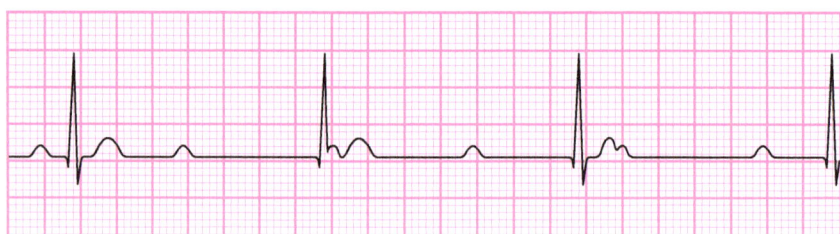

Third-degree heart block
Mobitz type I

Bundle branch blocks

Bundle branch blocks occur when there's a delay or obstruction along the pathway that conducts electrical impulses to the ventricles. They can significantly alter the appearance of the QRS complex and usually make them wider on an ECG.

Right bundle branch block (RBBB): Characterized by a widened QRS complex (>0.12 seconds), with a distinctive "rabbit ear" appearance in leads V1 and V2.

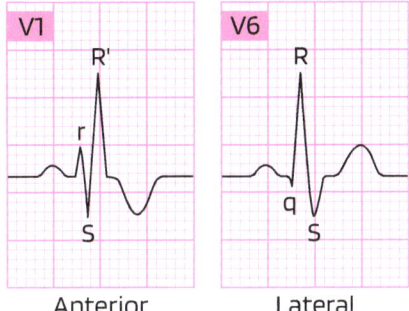

Right bundle branch block

Left bundle branch block (LBBB): Also presents with a widened QRS complex, accompanied by broad, notched R waves in leads I, aVL, V5, and V6, and deep S waves in leads V1 and V2.

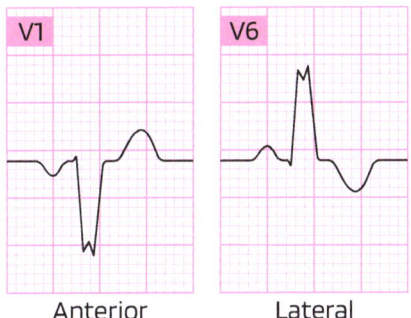

Left bundle branch block

Sick sinus syndrome (SSS)

In Sick Sinus Syndrome (SSS), the SA node, which is the heart's natural pacemaker, doesn't function properly. This can result in a variety of rhythms that are too fast, too slow, alternating between the two, or asystole (cardiac arrest for a few seconds). Ischemic heart disease, age-related degeneration, and certain drugs are the most common causes.

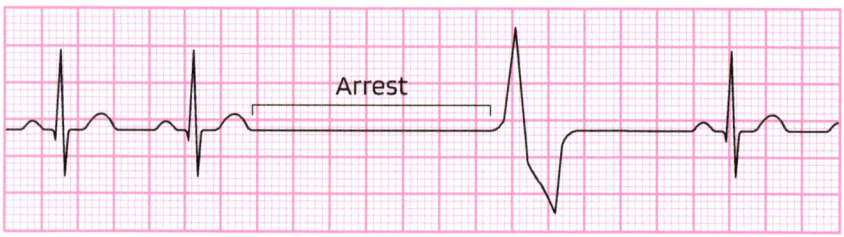

Arrest

Sick sinus syndrome

Long QT syndrome

Long QT syndrome (LQTS) is a disorder of myocardial repolarization characterized by an elongated QT interval on the ECG. It increases the risk of sudden cardiac death due to torsades de pointes, a form of polymorphic ventricular tachycardia.

ECG findings: A QT interval that, when corrected for heart rate (QTc), exceeds 470 ms in men and 480 ms in women.

Management: Avoiding QT-prolonging medications, maaning electrolytes, and in some cases, the use of beta-blockers or an implantable cardioverter-defibrillator (ICD) are indicated.
Since the QT interval shortens at higher heart rates and lengthens at lower heart rates, it's often corrected for heart rate to provide a standardized value known as the corrected QT interval (QTc).

A commonly used formula to correct the QT interval for heart rate is Bazett's formula:

QTc =QT/(√RR)

Where:
> QTc is the corrected QT interval,
> QT is the measured QT interval from the ECG,
> RR is the interval between two consecutive R-waves, measured in seconds (this is essentially the inverse of the heart rate).

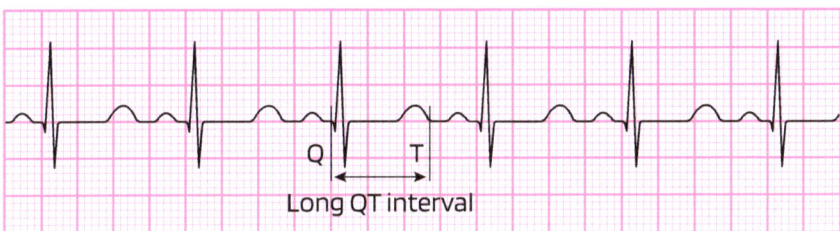

Q   T
Long QT interval

Long QT syndrome

The pre-excitation syndromes

Pre-excitation syndromes, such as Wolff-Parkinson-White (WPW) syndrome, involve an abnormal accessory electrical pathway that bypasses the normal conduction system, leading to premature ventricular activation.

ECG characteristics:
> Short PR interval.
> Widened QRS complex.
> Delta wave (a slurred upstroke in the QRS complex).

Clinical implications: Patients with pre-excitation syndromes may experience episodes of supraventricular tachycardia and are at risk for other arrhythmias. They may experience palpitations, dizziness or syncope.

Both risk of atrial fibrillation and sudden cardiac death are increased in WPW.

Management

Beta blockers or calcium channel blockers can be used in the management of WPW.

Catheter ablation can destroy the accessory pathway be using radiofrequency energy.

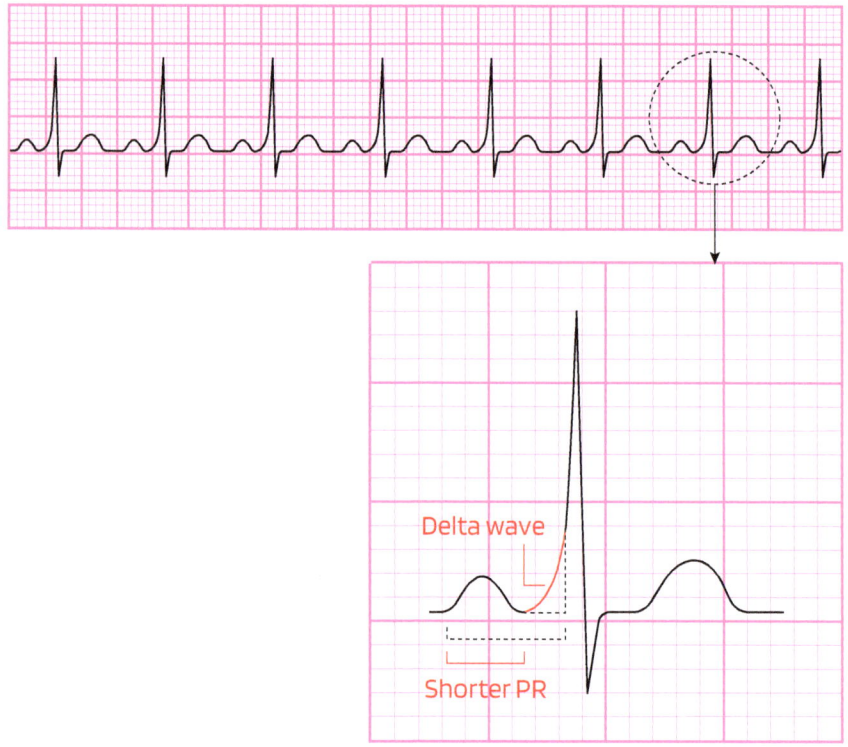

Wolf-Parkinson-White sydnroeme

Chapter 4
Ischemic heart disease

Ischemic heart disease and ECG

Ischemic heart disease (IHD) results from reduced blood flow to the heart muscle, often due to atherosclerosis. ECG findings in IHD may include:

> **ST-segment elevation:** Indicative of acute myocardial infarction (AMI), where there is a complete blockage of blood flow to a part of the heart.

> **ST-segment depression:** Suggestive of myocardial ischemia, a condition where the heart muscle is receiving insufficient blood flow.

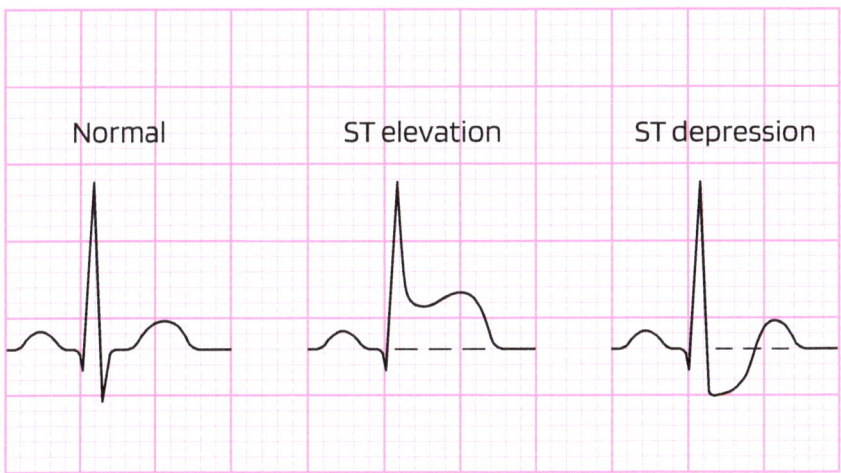

ST elevation and ST depression

> **T-wave inversion:** This can also indicate ischemia or may be a sign of a recent myocardial infarction (MI).

> **Q wave:** The presence of a Q wave on an ECG can indicate a previous myocardial infarction. Pathological Q waves are deep and wide and suggest that there has been significant myocardial necrosis.

In the context of an acute or new infarct, smaller Q waves may begin to appear and signify the onset of myocardial necrosis.

Myocardial Infarction:
Recognizing patterns and localizing MI

Myocardial infarction (MI) presents distinct ECG patterns depending on the infarct's location. Recognizing these patterns is crucial for timely intervention.

ECG not only allows for the detection of an MI but also for the localization of the affected area, guiding treatment decisions.

Wall	Artery	Leads
Septal	LAD	V1 – V2
Anterior	LAD	V2 – V4
Anteroseptal	LAD	V1 – V4
Lateral	LCA	I, aVL
Anterolateral	LAD and/or LCA	V3 – V6 (I, aVL maybe present)
Inferior	RCA	II, III, aVF
Extensive anterolateral	Left main	V2 – V6 and I, aVL Reciprocal changes in II, III, aVF maybe seen
Posterior	PDA (Posterior descending artery)	V1 – V3 (tall R with ST depression)

Localization of the myocardial infarction

Lateral wall myocardia infarction

Lateral M is diagnosed by ST elevation in leads I and aVL, V5 and/ or , and V6.

The presence of ST depression in the inferior wall leads can by the reciproacal chanes or lateral wall myocareia infarction.

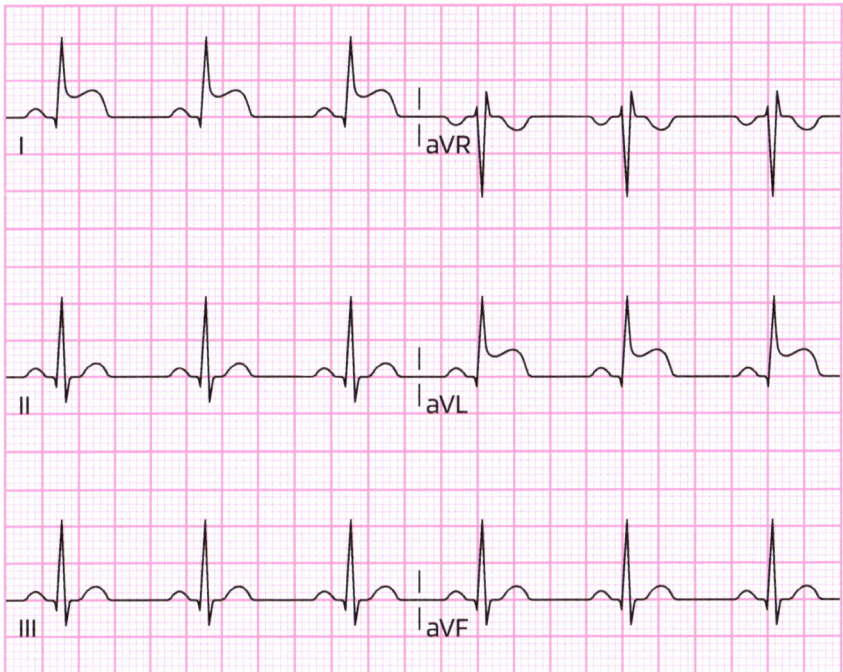

Lateral wall myocardial infarction

Inferior wall myocardial infarcation

Inferior wall MI is diagnosed by seeing ST elevation in leads II, III, and aVF.

ST depression in lateral leads lead I and aVL) can be seen in inferior wall MI which is just the reciprocal changes.

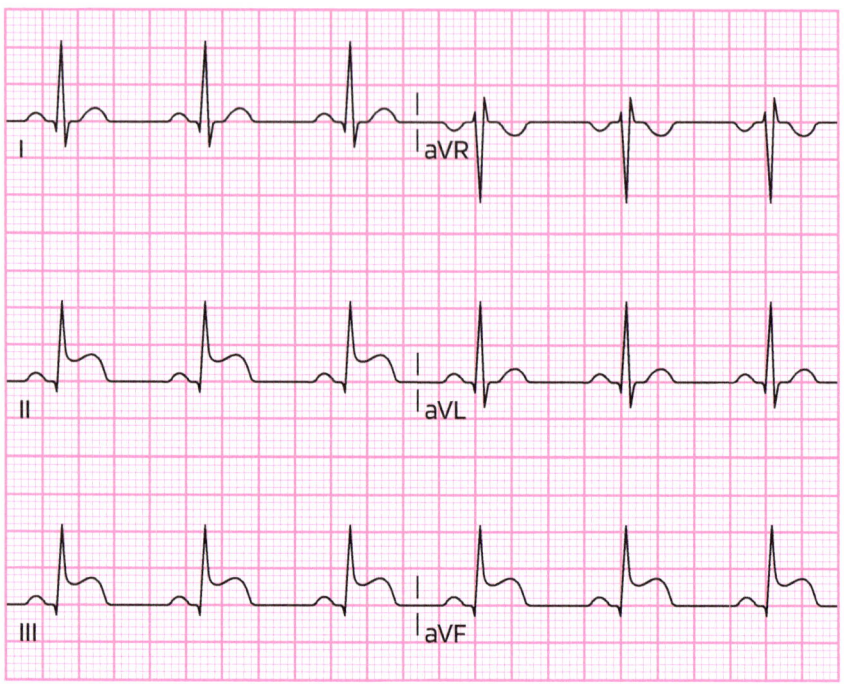

Inferior wall myocardial infarction

Left main coronary artery myocardial infarcation

Diagnosis of left main coronary artery MI is very important since the management is mostly surgical.

The ECG findings include significant ST–segment elevation in multiple leads, especially in the precordial leads (V2–V6), indicating widespread ischemia or injury. ST elevation can also appear in leads I and aVL, since left circuflex artery is a branch of left main coronary artery.

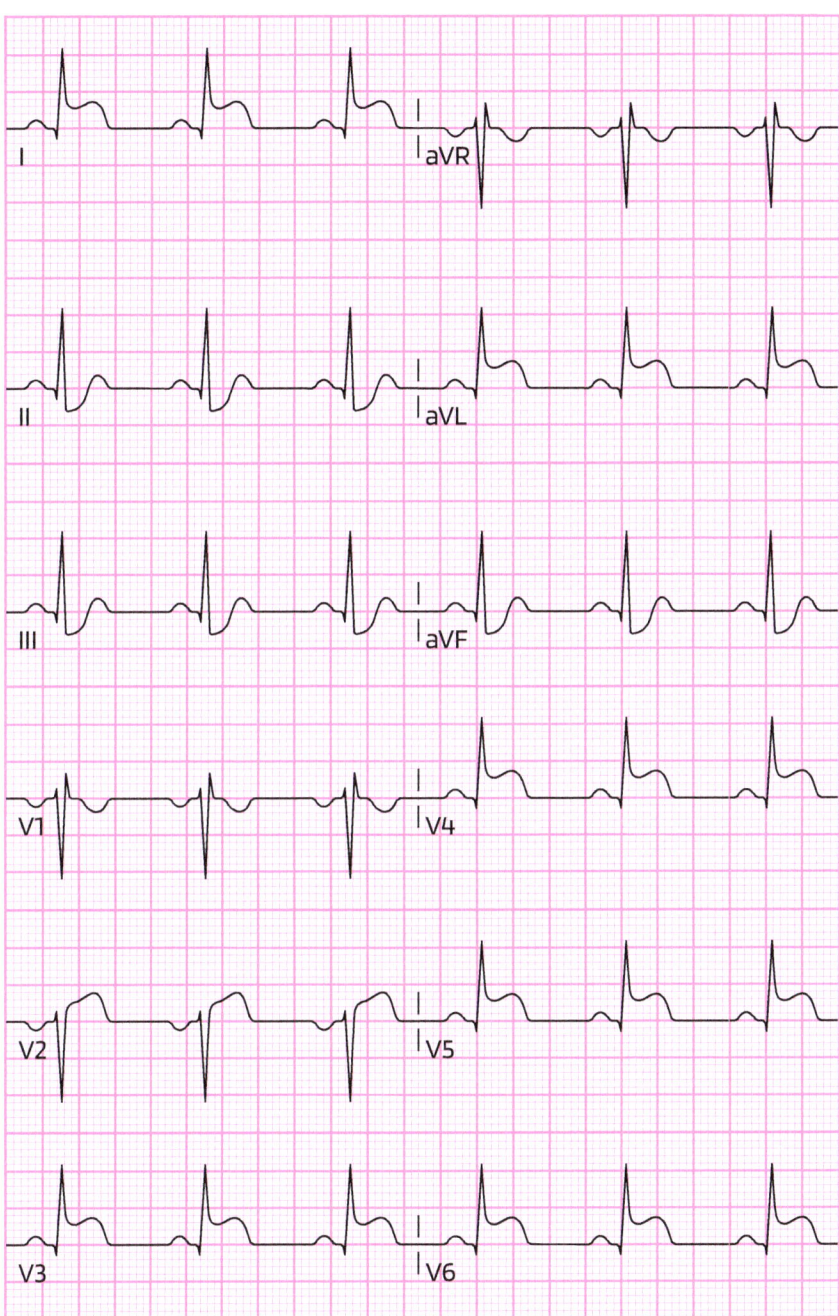

Left main coronary artery myocardial infarction

Anterolateral wall myocardial infarction

ST-segment elevations are typically seen in the anterior (V3, V4) and lateral leads (I, aVL, V5, V6).

Posterior wall MI

ST depression in the anterior leads with tall R waves, may be a sign of posterior wall MI, requiring additional posterior leads for confirmation.

Other conditions
Hypokalemia and U waves

Hyperkalemia may cause peaked T waves, while hypokalemia can lead to U waves and flattened T waves.

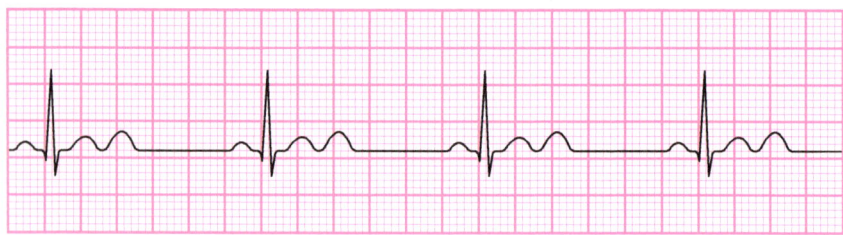

Hypokalemia and U wave

Hyperkalemia

Hyperkaelemia can present with peaked T waves.

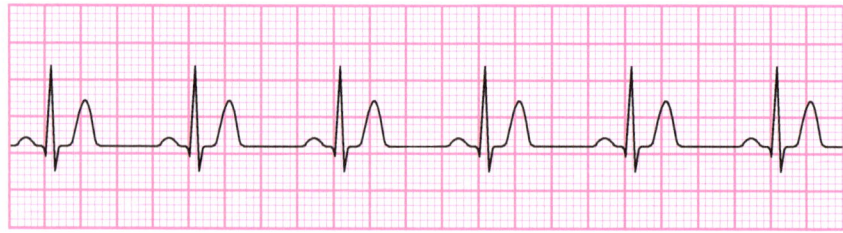

Tall T waves in hyperkalemia

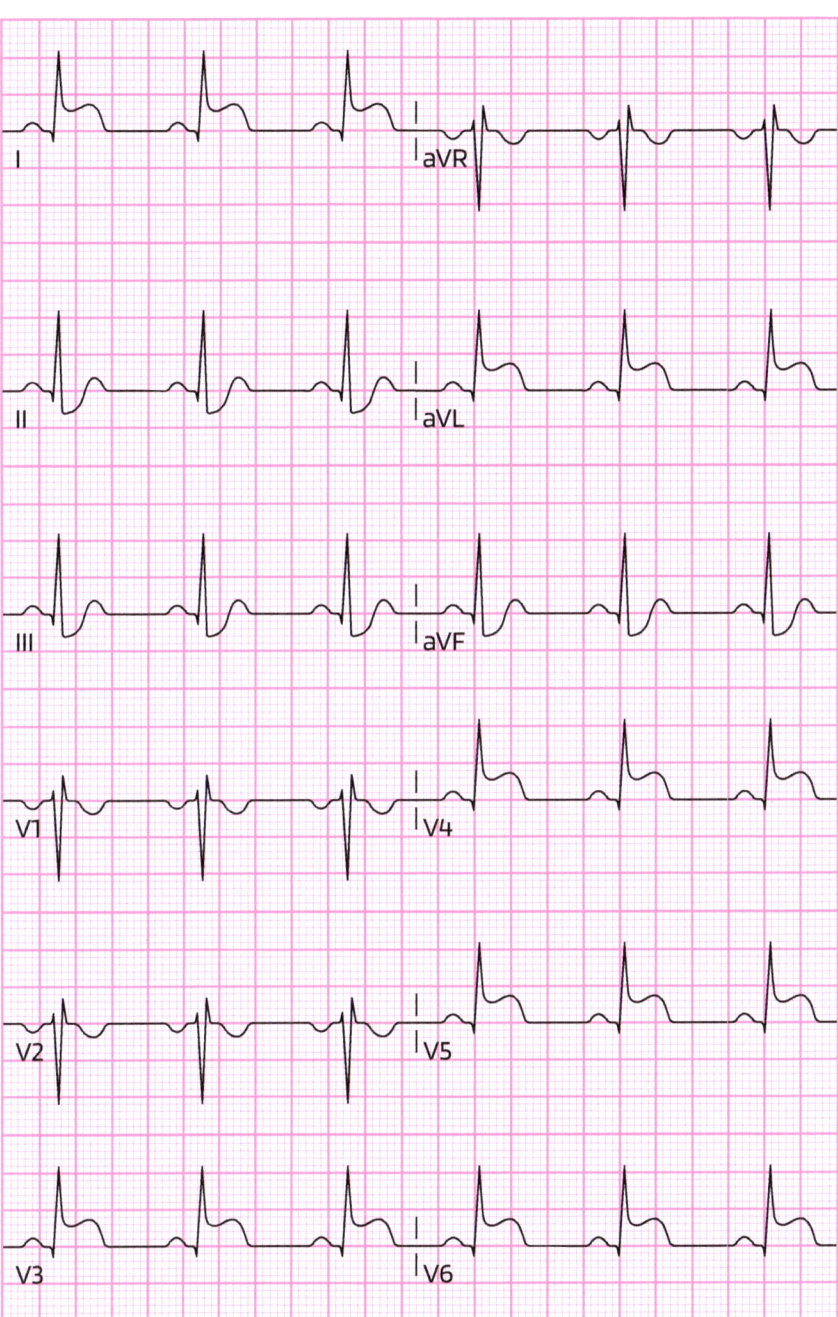

Anterolateral myocardial infarction

Pericarditis

Inflammation of the pericardium (pericarditis) often shows diffuse ST elevation and PR depression.

In many cases of pericarditis, pericardial effusion is present, characterized on ECG by beat-by-beat changes in the height of the QRS complex, known as electrical alternans. The ECG below shows electrical alternans, which are seen in pericardial effusion. As the fluid around the heart moves, the height of the QRS complex changes.

The strip below shows electrical alternans.

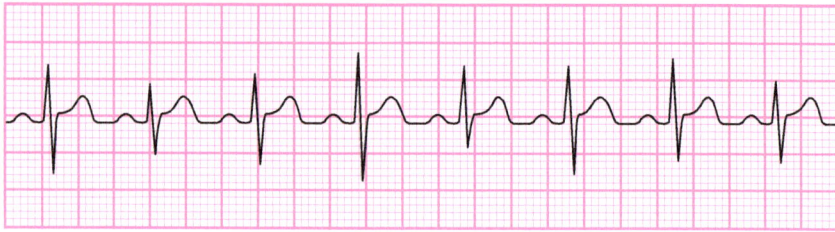

Pericarditis with electrical alternans

Pulmonary embolism

The most common finding is sinus tachycardia. Right axis deviation or right bundle branch block and T wave inversions can also be seen. **S1Q3T3** is a classic finding and includes a prominent S wave in lead I, a Q wave in lead III, and an inverted T wave in lead III. This pattern is considered a sign of acute right heart strain and is seen in only 15 percent of cases.

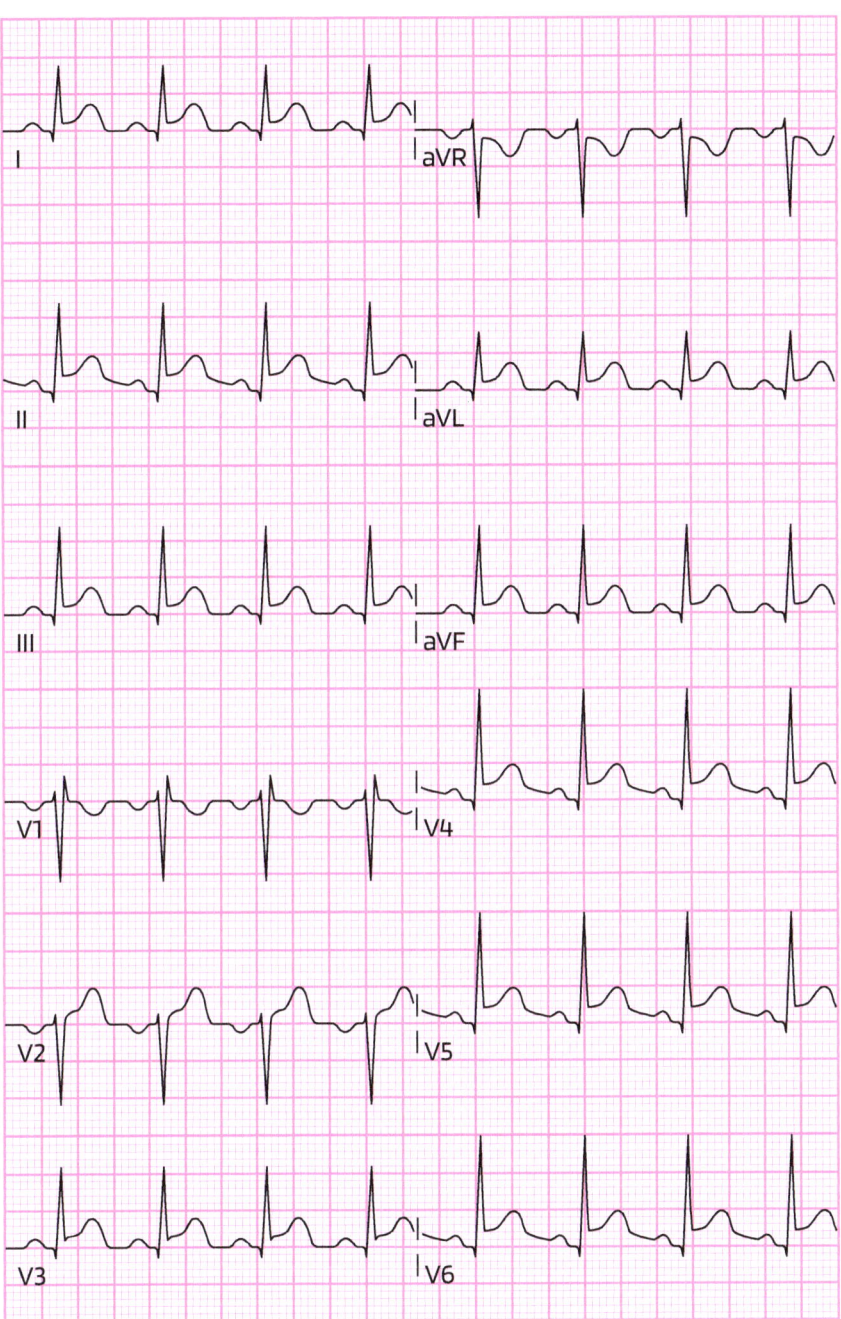

Pericarditis with diffuse ST elevation

Brugada syndrome

Characterized by a coved ST-segment elevation in leads V1 to V3, Brugada syndrome is associated with an increased risk of sudden cardiac death. This genetic disorder affects the heart's electrical system, potentially leading to dangerous arrhythmias. Early diagnosis and management are crucial to prevent life-threatening events.

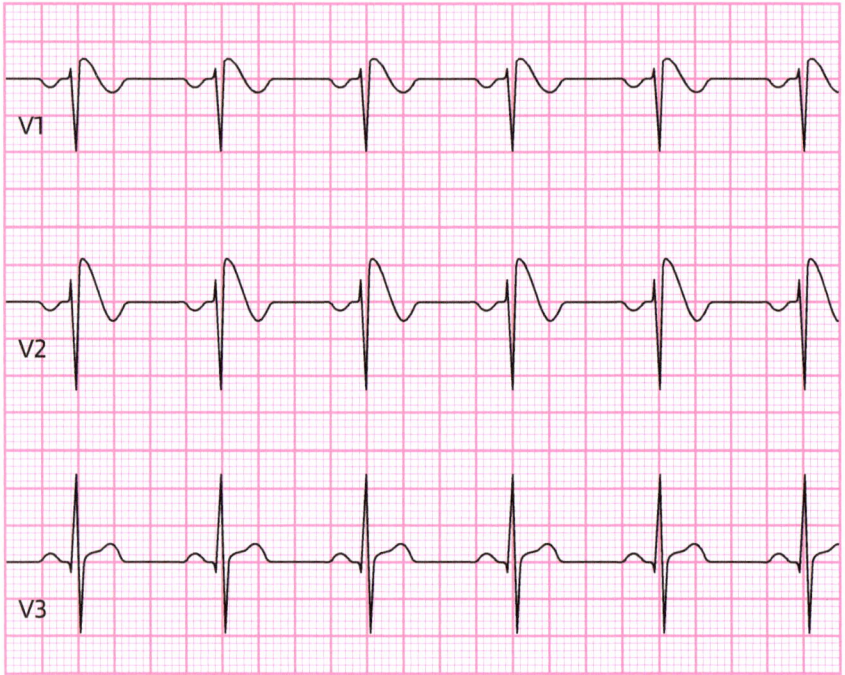

Brugada syndrome

Left ventricular aneurysm

An ECG showing a left ventricular aneurysm typically presents with persistent ST-segment elevation in leads corresponding to the aneurysm's location. This is often associated with deep, broad pathological Q waves, reflecting myocardial scarring.

This persistent elevation is unlike the transient ST elevation seen in acute MI.

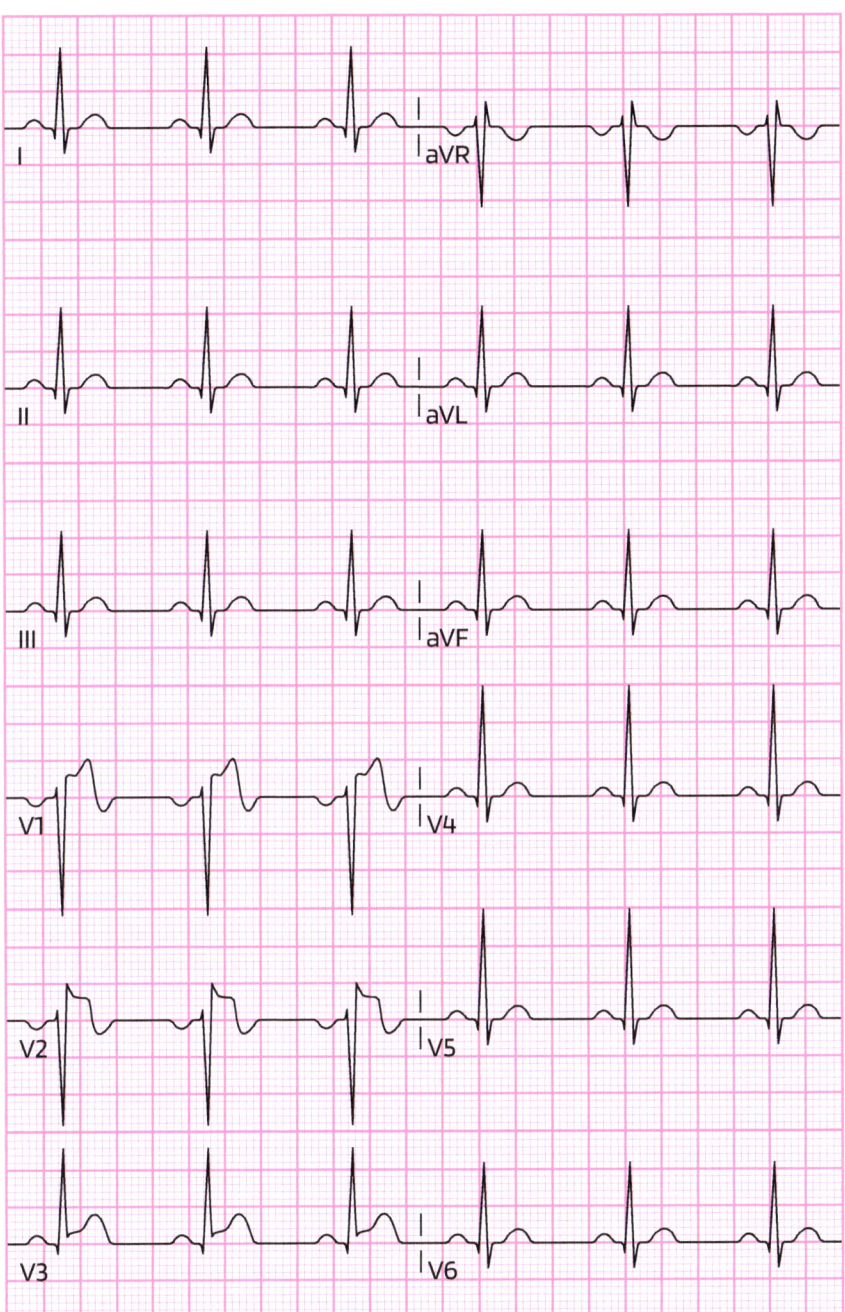

Left ventricular aneurysm